# ORAL DELIGHTS:
## UNLEASHING INTENSE PLEASURE AND CONNECTION THROUGH SEX

**Robert Matthes**

All rights reserved. No part of this publication may be reproduced, distributed, or transmitted in any form or by any means, including photocopying, recording, or other electronic or mechanical methods, without the prior written permission of the publisher, except in the case of brief quotations embodied in critical reviews and certain other noncommercial uses permitted by copyright law.

Copyright © (Robert Matthes), (2023).

# TABLE OF CONTENTS

# **INTRODUCTION**

People often attempt to mend relationships by centering their attention on the issues that exist inside them, but they do not begin with the fundamental (and maybe most essential) component of a committed partnership. Nothing of value can ever be constructed in the absence of trust.

A connection built on trust will last far longer than one that does not.

# CHAPTER 1

It is essential to begin from the very beginning by establishing a strong foundation of trust. If you give the impression of being difficult to get, date other people, or behave in any other manner that undermines trust, it may begin to damage the basis of the relationship, which can be difficult to restore in the future."

If you make an effort to be there for your spouse from the very beginning of your relationship, that pattern will continue to play out over the course of your time together. Be there as a support system for them, make yourself accessible to them, and be honest about how you're feeling. "You lay the groundwork for a solid foundation by acting in ways that let your partner know you are there for them and they can count on you." Although there are a lot of complex elements, the following list includes the elements that I believe are the most critical to building a solid foundation. "If you act in ways that let your partner know you are there for them and they can count on you, you lay the groundwork for a solid foundation." If these components are missing from your partnership, it is quite unlikely that you will be able to make any progress in improving the situation.

· Trust

· Commitment

· Appreciating one another is the key to putting an end to animosity.

· Being open and exposing oneself to risk

Open and honest communication.

# MAKE SURE TO ALLOW PLENTY OF TIME FOR CONVERSATIONS.

It is impossible to have a happy and healthy partnership without effective communication in the relationship. Because your significant other is typically the one with whom you spend the most time, there is a larger possibility of misunderstandings and arguments arising between the two of you.

But you will be rewarded for your efforts when you improve communication in your relationships.

It might be nerve-wracking to open up to another person about how we are feeling, but doing so is what sets apart our closest friendships from the acquaintances we meet at happy hour, and you want your relationship to be in the former group.

"Vulnerability starts to create the wall of trust, which will continue to pay off over the whole of the partnership," "Spend time together intentionally getting to know each other in a more profound way.

The establishment of a robust emotional connection may be facilitated by making time and providing a setting in which people can discuss their desires, anxieties, hopes, ambitions, emotions, objectives, values, and requirements.

We all know couples that seem to argue all the time, as well as couples who don't appear to argue at all. Both types of couples exist. Even though every partnership has its ups and downs, a lack of communication in a relationship is a red flag in any circumstance, including frequent fighting and no fighting at all. The important thing is not to avoid ever having a debate with your spouse.

It is to enhance your abilities at conflict resolution by applying the eight ideas that were presented above so that when conflicts do occur, you will be able to transform them into something that enriches your relationship rather than something that weakens it.

## FRIENDSHIP WITH THE PERSON YOU ARE INVOLVED WITH

We know that good closeness in a relationship is established via the forging of solid friendships between the partners, and a strong long-term relationship goes deeper than just physical desire. "Knowing one another, showing affection and appreciation for one another, and being receptive to one another's need for connection and attention are all essential components of friendship.

## CONTRIBUTIONS

When we are enthusiastic about a new romantic connection, it is simple for us to make all of the necessary preparations and put in all of the necessary work without even recognizing it. It is crucial to make sure that both partners are participating equally, despite the fact that we don't want to play any games.

Relationships are work, and you need to give the one(s) you're in the midst of the same degree of consideration and attention that you do to your job. Maintaining consistent communication with your spouse to find out how they are feeling on an emotional level is important because it provides you both with the chance to bring up concerns before they become a problem.

Establishing these check-ins at an early stage will set the stage for a prosperous future for your partnership. "Creating room for a conversation about business can be helpful in reducing feelings of anxiety or uncertainty,"

"It's important to be able to openly express your admiration for one another," It is simpler for us to be vulnerable and personal in a relationship when we feel liked and valued by the other person.

If your time in bed with your spouse isn't all you'd want it to be, it may be worth investigating some new methods to rejuvenate things. Having a date night with your lover to remind yourself of all the reasons you admire each other and to relax by getting wined and fed may be nice, Of course, there may be a medical reason why your sexual life is declining. Diabetes, thyroid difficulties, cancer, and heart problems might reduce sexual drive. Nerve difficulties or other abnormalities may cause sex to be unpleasant for women. And some drugs include those for blood pressure, depression, and anxiety. That's why it's crucial to obtain a medical examination if you are having symptoms that disrupt your sexual life and have your disease appropriately handled. You may also ask your doctor whether it's possible to switch your prescription to one without a sexual adverse effect.

# CHAPTER 2

## Making Sex a Priority

Sometimes, having more and better sex just means clearing your calendar. "It's hard to be in the mood when you have a million things on your to-do list and not much time to accomplish them. In this day of being always busy, sometimes we need to create the time instead of simply spontaneously assuming things like sex will find time for them. Set your alarm 30 minutes early, or go to bed purposely early. By segmenting time expressly for sex, you'll never merely forget, as well as offer yourself a chance to look forward to it." Of course, we're not advising you to have sex if you don't want to. But definitely try dipping your toe into some sexual activity, even if you don't believe you're in the mood. Sometimes our bodies are up for it even though our minds aren't. This is especially true for women, who often need some stimulation to create arousal rather than the other way around. "Prioritising sex means getting it whenever you can."

A quickie in the shower, a hand job before your yoga class

If you want to make sex a priority, sometimes you have to be open to taking what you can get!"

"When couples become too preoccupied with orgasm-focused, penetrative sex, anxiety can cloud their experience. They start chasing orgasms and block their ability to experience pleasure not directly related to the end game." This might turn some partners off entirely if they believe they can't perform to the point of orgasm.

They may wonder, Why bother? So you can see why putting fun first without constantly stressing about the aim of coming is crucial.

Make a point of thinking about you and your partner getting hot and heavy throughout your commute or while at work. "These fantasies keep your sexy 'pilot light' burning even when the realities of life prevent you from indulging as often as you'd like".

# SEX POSITIONS FOR ORGASM IN WOMEN

Just like adopting better-for-you food and exercise habits, getting into the habit of having more (and better) sex will require time and effort until it always seems simple and natural. But your sexual health is equally as vital as your mental and physical health so don't disregard that aspect of yourself.

During sex, most women will tell you that climaxing increases pleasure. And let's be honest: bringing your spouse across the finish line makes you feel pretty good, too. The good news? Although porn may lead you to assume otherwise, you don't need to be hung like a horse or ploughed like a jackhammer in order for your partner to attain climax. Instead, if your spouse has a vulva, merely concentrate on particular postures that target two extremely sensitive erogenous zones: the clitoris and the G-spot. Of course, everyone's anatomy is somewhat unique, meaning what makes one person groan with pleasure can simply not work for another.

Observes that some cisgender women believe that clitoral touch is really too forceful during sex. That's why communication is crucial when trying out various positions.

Don't be scared to ask your spouse,

"Does that feel good?"

"Did you like it when I leaned forward more?" or "Want me to go slower or faster?" " The first third of the vaginal canal is most pleasure-prone as it is enmeshed in the clitoral structures, so interspersing slow shallow strokes with deeper strokes is bound for their pleasure; some pressure against the cervix also lights up the somatosensory cortex in the brain, along with clitoral and nipple stimulation." This implies that an optimal sex position to assist your spouse would involve clitoral consistency, breast stimulation, and occasional cervical touch.

• kneel and straddle their left leg while they're resting on their left side. From here, they should bend their right leg over the right side of your waist, allowing full access to their vagina.

# CHAPTER 3

This position is an enhancement over conventional missionary since it positions you up for deeper penetration and enables you to delay your roll. "With your partner on their side, the girth of your penis will be hitting and stressing their g-spot in novel ways while also enabling you to retain a clitoral connection, which is sometimes sacrificed in positions that promote g-spot stimulation. Spend some time examining their bodies. This configuration allows you complete access to their clitoris for manual stimulation. But don't feel constrained to only hands-on pleasure. Try withdrawing your penis and, while holding the shaft with your left hand, massaging the head on their clitoris. Start out nice and slow, then, as you build pace and pressure, reinsert once you've pushed them to the edge of an orgasm.

• Stand at the edge of a bed as your spouse leans back and lifts their legs to their chest. Their knees are bent as though they're undertaking a "bicycling" workout. Grab their ankles and penetrate them. You'll want to start by thrusting gently since the deep entry may be initially unpleasant. Have them position their heels on your shoulders, which will expand their hips so their labia rub against you. This posture is also ideal for manual clitoral stimulation.

• You and your partner lay down on your backs, facing the same direction, with one of you behind the other. Because your lover wants you to have better access to their vagina, they will bend their knees and pull their rear end toward you. The angle at which you enter will change depending on how you tilt your bodies, which will also aid with rocking and thrusting. You are able to reach around and play with their breasts from this vantage point. There is a possibility that you may manually stimulate their clitoris if you approach it from the right angle. Because you are in this posture, you may achieve both deep penetration and body touch.

• While they are lying on their backs, you should have them place their legs over your shoulders. The angle formed by their bodies needs to be close to ninety degrees. As a result of the fact that it enables deep vaginal penetration, this legs-on-shoulders action ought to be regarded as standard. If the traditional G-Whiz isn't doing anything for them, you may try grasping their buttocks and tilting their pelvis forward, a little toward you. This is an alternative to the G-Whiz.

Always be sure to ask them what feels best; a little adjustment might be the difference between them not orgasming at all and orgasming within a few minutes. A wonderful position for stimulating the clitoral and cervical regions as well as engaging in eye-to-eye lovemaking and achieving attunement, the supine posture you should gently hoist them up while your arms are wrapped over their neck and upper back. This not only allows them to get more penetration, but it also makes the experience seem more intense since it compels both of you to stare directly into the eyes of the other person.

• You've laid down and are now lying on your back. They place one leg on either side of your body and straddle you in this position.

There are a lot of different takes on the cowgirl, so it's important to discuss with your partner which version is going to be most enjoyable for them. It's possible that they find it more comfortable to have their feet planted on both sides of you, making it seem as if they are sitting on you rather than riding. They may like it since leaning back allows for deeper penetration, which may be one of the reasons why they do it.

They could like it when you do all the pushing, but in most cases, taking charge of the situation gives them the ability to have orgasms more quickly. They are the ones who choose the tempo, how far you should delve, and which perspectives you should approach from.

They are able to provide themselves with all they need to have an orgasmic experience when they are in charge. You may continue grinding your penis against your spouse even while your tumescence (erection) is fading, which is a huge benefit for males who come first in the relationship.

• They begin by sitting on their heels and gradually go into a forward-leaning position. They continue to sit on their haunches and reach their hands in front of them while maintaining a straight back throughout the whole movement. Let's speak about child's pose now that we've already started integrating yoga into our sexual practice. To begin, if they have a problem with their back, this posture is excellent for them since it elongates the muscles in their back. Even if they don't suffer from back discomfort, they'll find that this posture is really soothing. Because of this, the neutral posture is often used in yoga when you need a break from completing other poses that are more taxing.

• Place them on the edge of the bed, assuming a position where they are standing on all fours. While you are standing behind them, instruct them to arch their backs in such a way that their buttocks are lifted skyward.

While maintaining your position with your legs outside of theirs, use your thighs to apply pressure to their knees, which pulls their vagina closer to your penis. This position is ideal for G-spot stimulation and also provides a wonderful view of their curves. "It's the squeeze of the knees together that will provide pleasurable friction against your penis and stimulation of the vestibular bulbs that are part of the clitoris and press against the vagina at the entrance."

• Have them lie on their stomachs on the bed with their knees bent slightly and their hips elevated slightly in the position shown. You may want to propose that they place a cushion beneath their lower abdominals for comfort as well as to improve the angle of their hips.

From where you are, approach them from behind and hold yourself up using your arms to keep your weight off of them as you go forward. This posture results in a close fit, which increases their enjoyment by giving them the impression that you are larger in size. "This is a great position for increasing your friction, achieving full penetration, and stimulating their g-spot all at the same time."

If you change your form such that you are thrusting less deeply and breathing more deeply, you will be able to hold this posture for a longer period of time.

## LUBRICATION IS THE BASIS OF COMMUNICATION.

Lubrication comes from good communication! In the event that you have never heard the proverb before, it is important to comprehend what it indicates.

The most important factor in having sexual encounters that are both pleasurable and beneficial to your health is to have an honest and open line of communication with your partner. There needs to be an open discourse about what you enjoy, what you don't like, what your limits are, and what sort of aftercare you want, and there ought to also be the opportunity to communicate during the act without the worry of "ruining the mood."

This conversation has to be open, honest, and devoid of any kind of judgement.

A safer sexual environment, which can only lead to better sex and a better relationship, may be created by being honest with your partner and listening to their needs in return.

When one or both couples are having any kind of pelvic floor dysfunction, it is very important to communicate with one another since the requirements of each partner will vary as a result of the condition.

Do not make them feel bad about their symptoms or their disorder. Encourage them to seek professional help and support them on their journey towards recovery.

Ask them how to make intimacy more comfortable and pleasurable.

- Do reassure them.

- Do communicate boundaries.

- Do not be afraid to seek counselling.

- Do not pressure or rush them.

- Do not take their symptoms personally.

- Do not make them feel bad about their symptoms or their disorder.

- Do not make them feel bad about their symptoms or their disorder.

Do not make them feel bad about their symptoms or their disorder.

• Do make sure that you are having a good time by using lubricant, toys, foreplay, and exploring other things outside of simple penetration!

Having pelvic floor dysfunction may be an emotionally trying, stressful, and tiring experience, and it is crucial for their spouse to be a source of love and support for them during these times. If you are the one who is experiencing pelvic discomfort or dysfunction, then it is your responsibility to be straightforward and honest about what it is that you need. It's not simple or convenient to speak about, but cooperating with one another is very necessary in order to make the experience of intimacy pleasurable for everyone involved. Without clear and open lines of communication, maintaining a healthy sexual life is almost impossible.

www.ingramcontent.com/pod-product-compliance
Lightning Source LLC
Chambersburg PA
CBHW072329270726
48658CB00016B/2227